Essential Dash Diet Slow Cooker Soups and Stews Recipes

Always New Delicious and Healthy Meals

Carmela Rojas

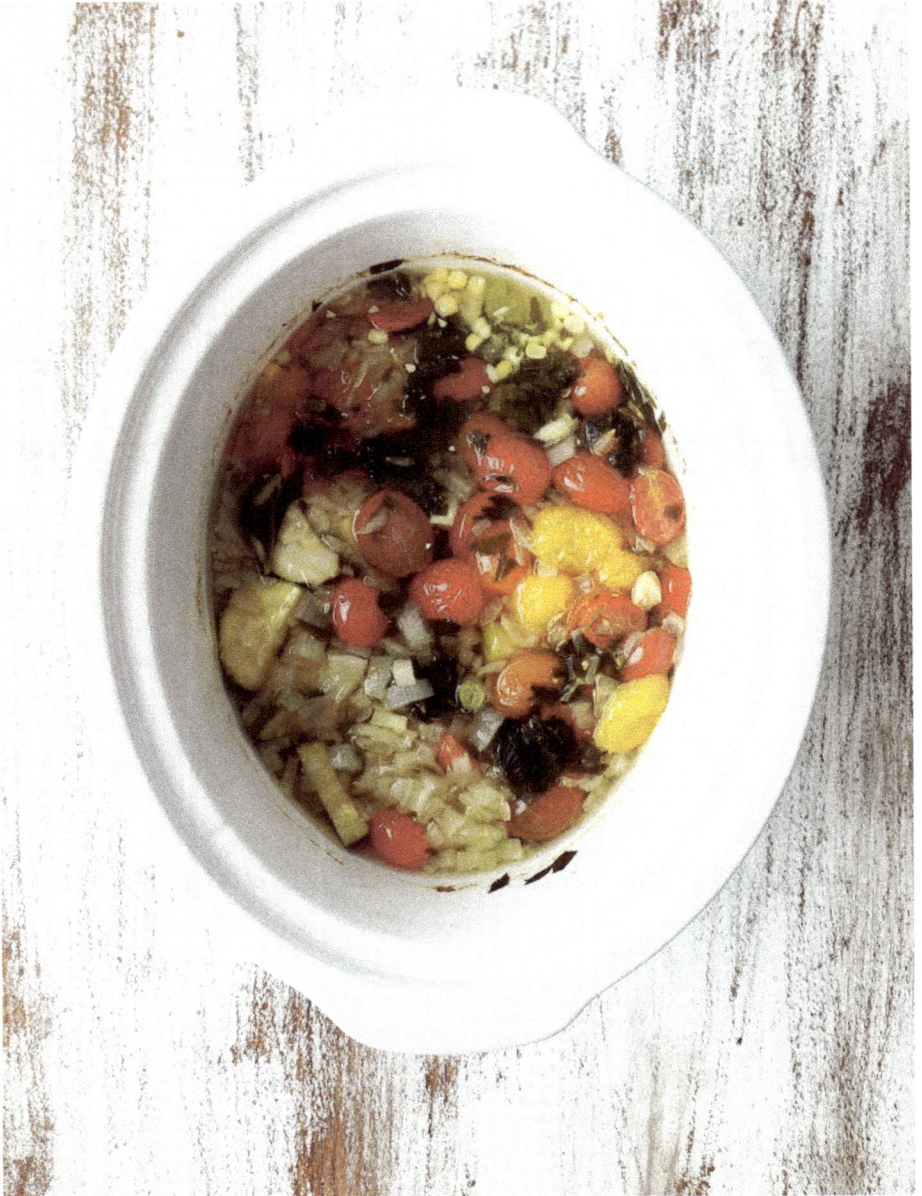

TABLE OF CONTENTS

5

Summer Vegetable Soup

Servings: 8 Servings

Ingredients:

- 4 cups (950 ml) low-sodium vegetable broth
- 8 ounces (225 g) frozen corn
- ½ cup (65 g) chopped carrots
- 8 ounces (225 g) frozen green beans
- 1 cup (120 g) sliced zucchini
- 2 cups (360 g) chopped tomatoes
- ½ cup (80 g) chopped onions
- ½ teaspoon minced garlic
- ½ teaspoon thyme
- ½ teaspoon basil
- ¼ teaspoon black pepper
- 1 cup (71 g) chopped broccoli
- ½ cup (65 g) frozen peas

Directions:

1. Combine all ingredients except broccoli and peas in slow cooker. Cover and cook on low 7 hours or on high 3½ hours. Stir in broccoli. Cook an additional 45

minutes on high. Stir in peas. Cook an additional 15 minutes on high.

Nutrition Info:

Per serving: 248 g water; 81 calories (12% from fat, 24% from protein, 65% from carb); 5 g protein; 1 g total fat; 0 g saturated fat; 0 g monounsaturated fat; 0 g polyunsaturated fat; 14 g carb; 4 g fiber; 3 g sugar; 101 mg phosphorus; 68 mg calcium; 1 mg iron; 120 mg sodium; 426 mg potassium; 2097 IU vitamin A; 1 mg ATE vitamin E; 30 mg vitamin C; 0 mg cholesterol

Curried Lima Soup

Servings: 6 Servings

Ingredients:

- 1½ cups (303 g) dried lima beans
- 4 cups (950 ml) water, divided
- 5 medium potatoes, finely chopped
- 2 cups (460 g) fat-free sour cream
- 2 tablespoons (13 g) curry powder

Directions:

1. In a medium saucepan, bring dried limas to a boil in 2 cups (475 ml) water. Boil, uncovered, for 2 minutes. Cover, turn off heat, and wait 2 hours. Drain water. Place beans in slow cooker. Add remaining 2 cups (475 ml) fresh water. Cover and cook 2 hours on high. During the last hour of cooking, add diced potatoes. Cook until potatoes are tender. Ten minutes before serving, add sour cream and curry powder.

Nutrition Info:

Per serving: 504 g water; 378 calories (24% from fat, 12% from protein, 64% from carb); 11 g protein; 11 g total fat; 6 g saturated

fat; 3 g monounsaturated fat; 1 g polyunsaturated fat; 62 g carb; 9 g fiber; 4 g sugar; 322 mg phosphorus; 142 mg calcium; 4 mg iron; 70 mg sodium; 1722 mg potassium; 417 IU vitamin A; 81 mg ATE vitamin E; 30 mg vitamin C; 31 mg cholesterol

Tuna And Red Pepper Stew

Servings: About 6

Cooking Time: 4 Hrs 15 Mins

Ingredients:

- 1 tbsp. Olive Oil
- 1 chopped Onion
- 1 minced clove Garlic
- ½ cup White Wine (dry)
- ¼ tsp. Pepper Flakes (red)
- 14 ounce diced Tomatoes
- 1 tsp. Paprika
- 1 pound scrubbed red potatoes
- 2 sliced roasted Bell Peppers (red)
- 2 pounds f Tuna Fillet
- 3 tbsp. Cilantro (chopped)

Directions:

1. Except for paprika, tuna and peppers, place all the ingredients in the slow cooker and cook on "high" for 2 hrs.
2. Add paprika, tuna, and peppers.
3. Cook again on "high" for 2 hrs.

4. Garnish with cilantro.

5. Serve hot.

Nutrition Info:

(Estimated Amount Per Serving): 107 Calories; 3 g Total Fat; 8 mg Cholesterol; 200 mg Sodium; 15 mg Carbohydrates; 2 g Dietary Fiber; 5 g Protein

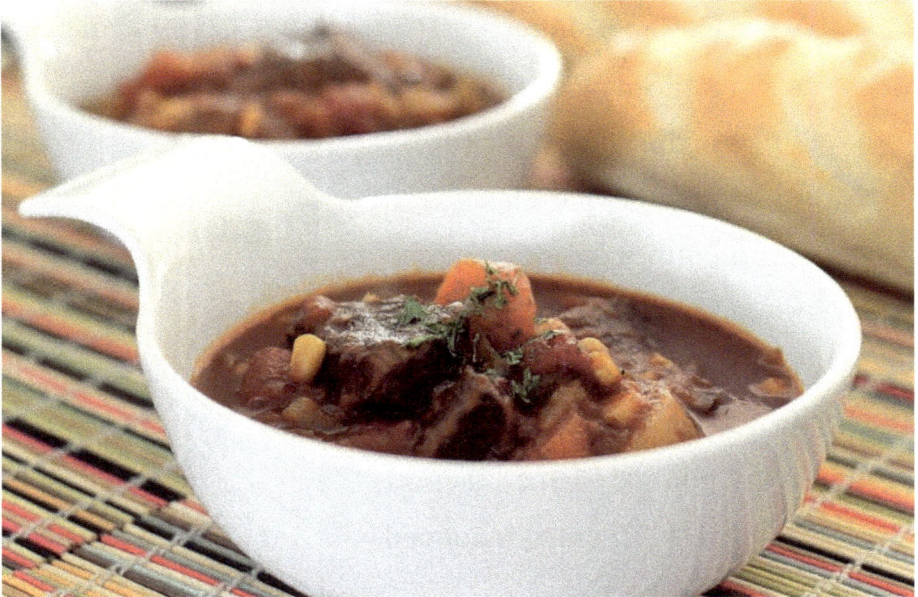

Easy Hamburger Soup

Servings: 6 Servings

Ingredients:

- 3 cups (700 ml) low-sodium beef broth
- 1 cup (100 g) chopped celery
- 2 cups (360 g) no-salt-added diced tomatoes
- 10 ounces (280 g) frozen mixed vegetables
- 1 cup (160 g) chopped onion
- 1 cup (130 g) sliced carrots
- 1 teaspoon pepper
- 1½ pounds (680 g) lean ground beef
- ½ cup (63 g) flour
- ½ cup (60 ml) water

Directions:

1. Combine all ingredients except flour and water in slow cooker. Cover and cook on low for 8 hours. One hour before serving time, turn to high. Add flour to water and stir until smooth. Pour into pot and stir. Cook until thickened, about 1 hour.

Nutrition Info:

Per serving: 384 g water; 378 calories (48% from fat, 28% from protein, 24% from carb); 26 g protein; 20 g total fat; 8 g saturated fat; 9 g monounsaturated fat; 1 g polyunsaturated fat; 22 g carb; 4 g fiber; 6 g sugar; 245 mg phosphorus; 74 mg calcium; 4 mg iron; 202 mg sodium; 781 mg potassium; 5793 IU vitamin A; 0 mg ATE vitamin E; 13 mg vitamin C; 78 mg cholesterol

Turkey Mushroom Soup

Servings: 8 Servings

Ingredients:

- ½ pound (225 g) ground turkey
- ½ teaspoon garlic powder
- ½ teaspoon onion powder
- ½ teaspoon black pepper
- ¼ cup (60 ml) egg substitute
- 1 tablespoon (15 ml) olive oil
- 1 cup (130 g) sliced carrots
- ½ teaspoon crushed garlic
- 2 cups (140 g) sliced mushrooms
- 2 cups (475 ml) low-sodium beef broth
- 10 ounces (280 g) low-sodium cream of mushroom soup
- 2 tablespoons (32 g) no-salt-added tomato paste

Directions:

1. In a small bowl, mix together ground turkey, garlic powder, onion powder, and pepper. Add egg substitute, stirring until well blended. Form into small meatballs. Heat olive oil in skillet. Brown meatballs

and drain well. Transfer meatballs to slow cooker. Add remaining ingredients. Cover and cook on low 6 to 8 hours or on high 3 to 4 hours.

Nutrition Info:

Per serving: 148 g water; 108 calories (35% from fat, 42% from protein, 23% from carb); 11 g protein; 4 g total fat; 1 g saturated fat; 2 g monounsaturated fat; 1 g polyunsaturated fat; 6 g carb; 1 g fiber; 2 g sugar; 122 mg phosphorus; 28 mg calcium; 1 mg iron; 96 mg sodium; 429 mg potassium; 2784 IU vitamin A; 1 mg ATE vitamin E; 2 mg vitamin C; 23 mg cholesterol

Soup For The Day

Servings: About 8

Cooking Time: 10 Hrs 10 Mins

Ingredients:

- 1 Beef Steak (cubed)
- 1 chopped Onion (med.)
- 1 tbsp. Olive Oil
- 5 thinly sliced med. Carrots
- 4 cups Cabbage
- 4 diced Red Potatoes
- 2 diced Celery Stalks
- 2 cans Tomatoes, diced
- 2 cans Beef Broth
- 1 tsp. Sugar
- 1 canTomato Soup
- 1 tsp.Parsley Flakes (dried)
- 2 tsp. Italian Seasoning

Directions:

1. In a skillet, sauté onion and steak in oil.
2. Transfer the sautéed mixture to the slow cooker.
3. Add rest of the ingredients to the slow cooker.

4. Cook on "low" for 10 hrs.

5. Serve hot.

Nutrition Info:

(Estimated Amount Per Serving): 259.6 Calories; 6.7 g Total Fat; 29.8 mg Cholesterol; 699.2 mg Sodium; 31.6 mg Carbohydrates; 4.6 g Dietary Fiber; 18.9 g Protein

Black Bean Soup

Servings: 8 Servings

Ingredients:

- 1 pound (455 g) dried black beans
- 2 cups (320 g) chopped onion
- 1 cup (150 g) chopped green bell pepper
- 1½ teaspoons minced garlic
- 1 tablespoon (7 g) cumin
- 2 teaspoons oregano
- 1 teaspoon thyme
- ½ teaspoon black pepper
- 3 cups (700 ml) water
- 2 tablespoons (28 ml) cider vinegar

Directions:

1. Soak beans overnight in water to cover. Drain. Combine beans and remaining ingredients in slow cooker. Cover and cook on low 8-10 hours.

Nutrition Info:

Per serving: 183 g water; 100 calories (5% from fat, 22% from protein, 73% from carb); 6 g protein; 1 g total fat; 0 g saturated

fat; 0 g monounsaturated fat; 0 g polyunsaturated fat; 19 g carb; 6 g fiber; 2 g sugar; 101 mg phosphorus; 44 mg calcium; 2 mg iron; 7 mg sodium; 318 mg potassium; 105 IU vitamin A; 0 mg ATE vitamin E; 18 mg vitamin C; 0 mg cholesterol

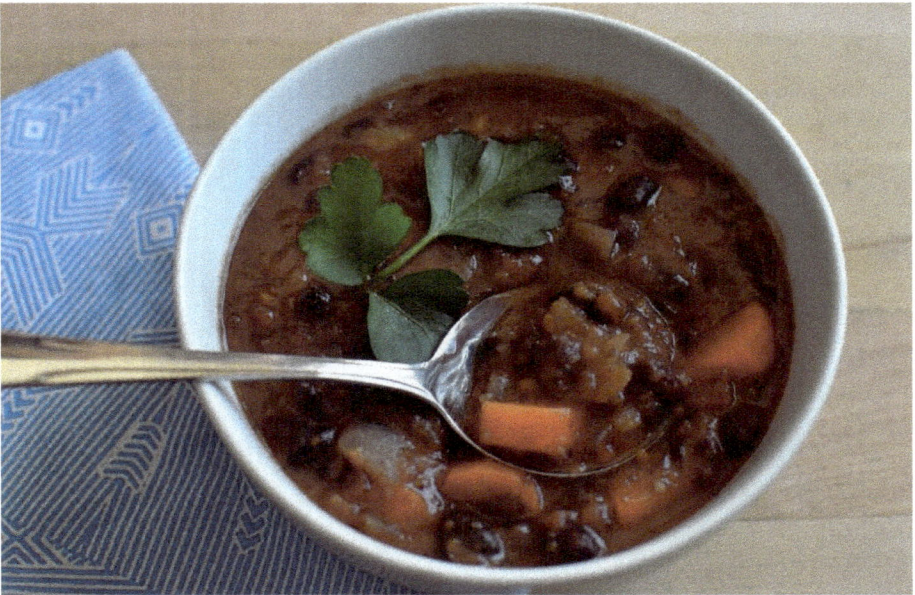

Pumpkin Soup

Servings: 6 Servings

Ingredients:

- ¼ cup (38 g) finely chopped green bell pepper
- ½ cup (80 g) finely chopped onion
- 1 cup (235 ml) low-sodium vegetable broth
- 2 cups (490 g) puréed pumpkin
- 2 cups (475 ml) skim milk
- ¼ teaspoon thyme
- ¼ teaspoon nutmeg

Directions:

1. Combine all ingredients in slow cooker and mix well. Cover and cook on low 5 to 6 hours.

Nutrition Info:

Per serving: 204 g water; 75 calories (8% from fat, 26% from protein, 65% from carb); 5 g protein; 1 g total fat; 0 g saturated fat; 0 g monounsaturated fat; 0 g polyunsaturated fat; 13 g carb; 3 g fiber; 3 g sugar; 138 mg phosphorus; 155 mg calcium; 1 mg iron; 77 mg sodium; 383 mg potassium; 12903 IU vitamin A; 50 mg ATE vitamin E; 10 mg vitamin C; 2 mg cholesterol

Beef Stew With Dumplings

Servings: 6 Servings

Ingredients:

- 1 pound (455 g) beef round roast, cubed
- 2 tablespoons (15 g) low-sodium onion soup mix
- 6 cups (1.4 L) low-sodium beef broth
- 1 cup (130 g) sliced carrot
- 2 potatoes, diced
- 1 cup (120 g) Heart-Healthy Baking Mix
- 1 tablespoon (1.3 g) parsley
- 6 tablespoons (90 ml) skim milk

Directions:

1. Place meat in cooker. Sprinkle with soup mix and then add broth and vegetables. Cover and cook on low for 6 to 8 hours. Combine baking mix, parsley, and milk. Drop by teaspoonfuls onto stew. Cover and cook on high until dumplings are done, 30 minutes to 1 hour.

Nutrition Info:

Per serving: 425 g water; 287 calories (11% from fat, 35% from protein, 54% from carb); 25 g protein; 4 g total fat; 2 g saturated fat; 2 g monounsaturated fat; 0 g polyunsaturated fat; 39 g carb; 3 g fiber; 2 g sugar; 344 mg phosphorus; 144 mg calcium; 4 mg iron; 341 mg sodium; 1085 mg potassium; 3731 IU vitamin A; 23 mg ATE vitamin E; 13 mg vitamin C; 43 mg cholesterol

Potato And Leek Soup

Servings: 6 Servings

Ingredients:

- 6 large potatoes, cubed
- 2 leeks, washed and cut up
- ½ cup (80 g) chopped onion
- ½ cup (65 g) grated carrot
- ¼ cup (25 g) chopped celery
- 1 tablespoon (1.3 g) parsley
- 5 cups (1.2 L) vegetable broth
- ¼ teaspoon pepper
- 1/3 cup (75 g) unsalted butter
- 13 ounces (370 ml) evaporated milk
- Chopped chives

Directions:

1. Put all ingredients into slow cooker or soup pot except milk and chives. Cook 10 to 12 hours on low or 4 to 6 hours on high. Stir in evaporated milk during last hour. To serve, sprinkle with chives.

Nutrition Info:

Per serving: 594 g water; 549 calories (32% from fat, 10% from protein, 58% from carb); 14 g protein; 20 g total fat; 11 g saturated fat; 6 g monounsaturated fat; 2 g polyunsaturated fat; 82 g carb; 8 g fiber; 6 g sugar; 418 mg phosphorus; 256 mg calcium; 4 mg iron; 224 mg sodium; 2076 mg potassium; 2922 IU vitamin A; 85 mg ATE vitamin E; 42 mg vitamin C; 45 mg cholesterol

Sausage And Bean Stew

Servings: 4 Servings

Ingredients:

- 1¼ cups (269 g) dried navy beans
- 1 pound (455 g) Italian sausage
- 1 cup (160 g) chopped onion
- ½ cup (50 g) sliced celery
- 1 cup (235 ml) dry red wine
- 1 teaspoon rosemary
- 1½ cups (355 ml) low-sodium vegetable broth
- 1 cup (180 g) chopped tomatoes

Directions:

1. Soak beans in water overnight. Drain, place in a pot, cover with water and simmer for 20 minutes. Drain. Place in slow cooker. Brown the sausage in a skillet over medium-high heat, stir in the onion and celery, and continue cooking until vegetables are soft. Place over the beans in the cooker. Combine remaining ingredients and pour over sausage-bean mixture. Cover and cook on high for 5 to 6 hours or low 8 to 10 hours.

Nutrition Info:

Per serving: 317 g water; 588 calories (63% from fat, 17% from protein, 20% from carb); 22 g protein; 38 g total fat; 13 g saturated fat; 17 g monounsaturated fat; 5 g polyunsaturated fat; 28 g carb; 7 g fiber; 3 g sugar; 301 mg phosphorus; 93 mg calcium; 3 mg iron; 130 mg sodium; 794 mg potassium; 295 IU vitamin A; 0 mg ATE vitamin E; 17 mg vitamin C; 86 mg cholesterol

Potato Soup

Servings: 8 Servings

Ingredients:

- 6 potatoes, peeled and diced
- 5 cups (1.2 L) low-sodium vegetable broth
- 2 cups (360 g) diced onion
- ½ cup (50 g) diced celery
- ½ cup (65 g) diced carrots
- ¼ teaspoon pepper
- 1½ cups (355 ml) evaporated milk
- 3 tablespoons (12 g) chopped fresh parsley

Directions:

1. Combine all ingredients except milk and parsley in slow cooker. Cover and cook on high 7 to 8 hours or until vegetables are tender. Stir in milk and parsley.

Nutrition Info:

Per serving: 452 g water; 296 calories (14% from fat, 16% from protein, 71% from carb); 12 g protein; 5 g total fat; 2 g saturated fat; 1 g monounsaturated fat; 1 g polyunsaturated fat; 54 g carb; 6 g fiber; 5 g sugar; 318 mg phosphorus; 201 mg calcium; 3 mg iron;

162 mg sodium; 1528 mg potassium; 1690 IU vitamin A; 2 mg ATE vitamin E; 30 mg vitamin C; 12 mg cholesterol

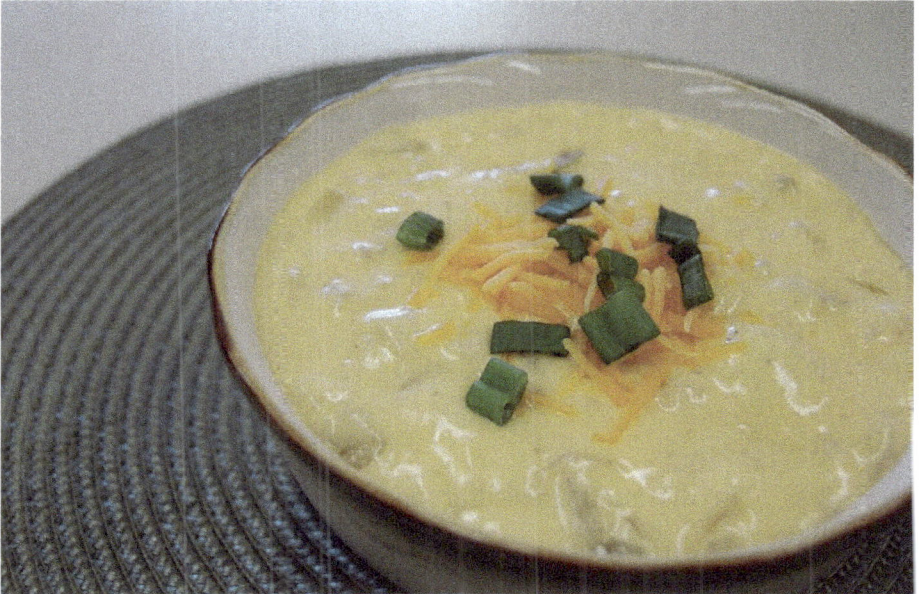

Alphabet Soup

Servings: 5 Servings

Ingredients:

- 1 pound (455 g) beef round roast, cubed
- 1 can (14 ounces, or 400 g) no-salt-added diced tomatoes
- 1 cup (245 g) no-salt-added tomato sauce
- 1 cup (235 ml) water
- 2 tablespoons (15 g) low-sodium onion soup mix
- 1 pound (455 g) frozen mixed vegetables
- ½ cup (75 g) alphabet pasta

Directions:

1. Brown meat in skillet over medium-high heat. Drain. Combine meat and remaining ingredients except pasta in slow cooker. Cover and cook on low 6 to 8 hours. Turn to high, add pasta, and cook until pasta is done, 30 minutes to 1 hour.

Nutrition Info:

Per serving: 307 g water; 290 calories (13% from fat, 38% from protein, 50% from carb); 27 g protein; 4 g total fat; 1 g saturated

fat; 1 g monounsaturated fat; 0 g polyunsaturated fat; 35 g carb; 6 g fiber; 7 g sugar; 316 mg phosphorus; 79 mg calcium; 4 mg iron; 106 mg sodium; 849 mg potassium; 4130 IU vitamin A; 0 mg ATE vitamin E; 16 mg vitamin C; 45 mg cholesterol

Fresh Vegetable Chili

Servings: 10 Servings

Ingredients:

- 1 tablespoon (15 ml) olive oil
- 1 cup (160 g) chopped onion
- 1 teaspoon minced garlic
- ½ cup (50 g) chopped celery
- ¾ cup (98 g) thinly sliced carrot
- 1 cup (150 g) chopped green bell pepper
- 1 cup (120 g) sliced zucchini
- 8 ounces (225 g) mushrooms, sliced
- 1¼ cups (285 ml) water
- 1 can (14 ounces, or 400 g) no-salt-added kidney beans, drained
- 1 can (14 ounces, or 400 g) no-salt-added diced tomatoes, undrained
- 1 teaspoon lemon juice
- ¼ teaspoon oregano
- 1 teaspoon ground cumin
- 1 teaspoon chili powder
- 1 teaspoon black pepper

Directions:

1. Heat oil in a skillet over medium heat; sauté onions and garlic until tender. Add celery, carrot, green pepper, zucchini, and mushrooms to skillet and sauté 2 to 3 minutes. Transfer to slow cooker. Add remaining ingredients. Cover and cook on low 6 to 8 hours.

Nutrition Info:

Per serving: 198 g water; 105 calories (14% from fat, 20% from protein, 65% from carb); 6 g protein; 2 g total fat; 0 g saturated fat; 1 g monounsaturated fat; 0 g polyunsaturated fat; 18 g carb; 6 g fiber; 5 g sugar; 115 mg phosphorus; 59 mg calcium; 2 mg iron; 49 mg sodium; 545 mg potassium; 7546 IU vitamin A; 0 mg ATE vitamin E; 23 mg vitamin C; 0 mg cholesterol

Chicken Vegetable Soup

Servings: 6 Servings

Ingredients:

- 1 can (28 ounces, or 785 g) no-salt-added diced tomatoes, undrained
- 2 cups (475 ml) low-sodium chicken broth
- 12 ounces (340 g) frozen corn
- ½ cup (50 g) chopped celery
- 1 can (6 ounces, or 170 g) no-salt-added tomato paste
- ¼ cup (48 g) lentils, rinsed
- 1 tablespoon (15 ml) Worcestershire sauce
- 1 teaspoon parsley flakes
- 1 teaspoon marjoram
- 1 cup (140 g) cubed cooked chicken breast

Directions:

1. Combine all ingredients in slow cooker except chicken. Cover and cook on low 6 to 8 hours. Stir in chicken 1 hour before the end of the cooking time.

Nutrition Info:

Per serving: 297 g water; 146 calories (9% from fat, 31% from protein, 60% from carb); 12 g protein; 2 g total fat; 0 g saturated fat; 0 g monounsaturated fat; 0 g polyunsaturated fat; 24 g carb; 5 g fiber; 9 g sugar; 163 mg phosphorus; 68 mg calcium; 3 mg iron; 144 mg sodium; 780 mg potassium; 651 IU vitamin A; 1 mg ATE vitamin E; 25 mg vitamin C; 20 mg cholesterol

Beef And Lentil Soup

Servings: 8 Servings

Ingredients:

- 1 pound (455 g) extra-lean ground beef
- 1 cup (160 g) chopped onion
- 2 potatoes, cubed
- 1 cup (130 g) sliced carrot
- 1 cup (100 g) sliced celery
- 1 cup (192 g) dry lentils
- 6 cups (1.4 L) low-sodium beef broth
- 1 can (14 ounces, or 400 g) no-salt-added diced tomatoes
- ½ teaspoon black pepper

Directions:

1. Brown meat in a nonstick skillet over medium-high heat. Drain. Combine meat and remaining ingredients in slow cooker. Cover and cook on low 8 to 10 hours.

Nutrition Info:

Per serving: 394 g water; 264 calories (35% from fat, 26% from protein, 38% from carb); 17 g protein; 10 g total fat; 4 g saturated

fat; 4 g monounsaturated fat; 1 g polyunsaturated fat; 26 g carb; 5 g fiber; 4 g sugar; 228 mg phosphorus; 60 mg calcium; 4 mg iron; 177 mg sodium; 978 mg potassium; 2814 IU vitamin A; 0 mg ATE vitamin E; 16 mg vitamin C; 39 mg cholesterol

Sweet Potato And Barley Stew

Servings: 6 Servings

Ingredients:

- 1 can (28 ounces, or 785 g) no-salt-added crushed tomatoes
- 1 medium sweet potato, peeled and cut into 1-inch (2.5 cm) cubes
- 2 cups (512 g) kidney beans, cooked or canned without salt
- 2 cups (475 ml) low-sodium chicken broth
- ½ cup (80 g) chopped onion
- ¾ cup (113 g) chopped red bell pepper
- ½ cup (100 g) pearl barley
- ½ cup (120 ml) water
- 1 tablespoon (7.5 g) chili powder
- 1 tablespoon (15 ml) lime juice
- 1 teaspoon minced garlic
- 1 teaspoon ground cumin
- ½ teaspoon oregano
- 1 teaspoon black pepper
- Lime wedges and/or chopped fresh cilantro (optional)

Directions:

1.   In a slow cooker, combine undrained tomatoes and remaining ingredients, except lime wedges and cilantro (if using). Cover and cook on low for 6 to 7 hours or on high for 3 to 4 hours. If desired, serve with lime wedges and/or top each serving with cilantro.

Nutrition Info:

Per serving: 316 g water; 190 calories (5% from fat, 20% from protein, 75% from carb); 10 g protein; 1 g total fat; 0 g saturated fat; 0 g monounsaturated fat; 0 g polyunsaturated fat; 38 g carb; 11 g fiber; 6 g sugar; 182 mg phosphorus; 98 mg calcium; 4 mg iron; 91 mg sodium; 723 mg potassium; 5088 IU vitamin A; 0 mg ATE vitamin E; 43 mg vitamin C; 0 mg cholesterol

Turkey Bean Soup

Servings: 12 Servings

Ingredients:

- 1 pound (455 g) ground turkey
- 1 cup (160 g) chopped onion
- 1 cup (100 g) sliced celery
- 2 cups (260 g) sliced carrot
- 4 cups (1 kg) kidney beans, cooked or canned without salt
- 4 cups (684 g) pinto beans, cooked or canned without salt
- 1 can (28 ounces, or 785 g) no-salt-added diced tomatoes
- 2 cups (475 ml) water
- 1 tablespoon (1.3 g) parsley
- 1 tablespoon (4 g) oregano
- 1 tablespoon (7 g) cumin

Directions:

1. Brown turkey and onions in skillet over medium-high heat. Combine turkey mixture and remaining

ingredients in slow cooker. Cover and cook on low 8 to 10 hours.

Nutrition Info:

Per serving: 212 g water; 389 calories (7% from fat, 32% from protein, 61% from carb); 32 g protein; 3 g total fat; 1 g saturated fat; 1 g monounsaturated fat; 1 g polyunsaturated fat; 60 g carb; 17 g fiber; 5 g sugar; 458 mg phosphorus; 152 mg calcium; 7 mg iron; 70 mg sodium; 1481 mg potassium; 3754 IU vitamin A; 0 mg ATE vitamin E; 14 mg vitamin C; 29 mg cholesterol

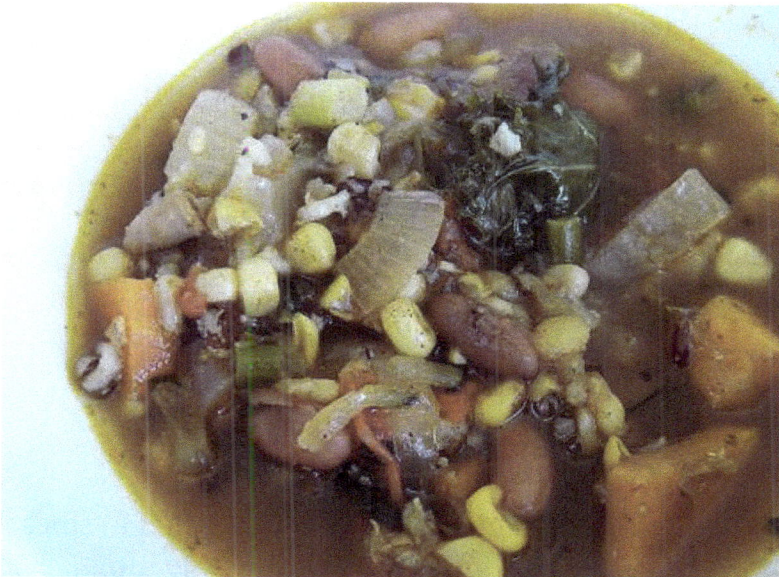

Lamb And Bean Stew

Servings: 6 Servings

Ingredients:

- 8 ounces (225 g) dried navy beans
- 6 cups (1.4 L) water
- 1 pound (455 g) lamb stew meat, cut into 1-inch (2.5 cm) cubes
- 4 cups (950 ml) low-sodium chicken broth
- 1 cup (130 g) carrots, cut into 1-inch (2.5 cm) pieces
- ½ cup (50 g) celery, cut into 1-inch (2.5 cm) pieces
- 1 onion, cut into wedges
- 1 cup (235 ml) dry white wine
- 2 teaspoons minced garlic
- 3 bay leaves
- 1½ teaspoons rosemary, crushed
- ¼ teaspoon black pepper

Directions:

1. Rinse and drain beans. In a 4-quart (3.8 L) stock pot, combine beans and the water. Bring to a boil; reduce heat and simmer for 10 minutes. Remove from heat. Cover and let stand for 1 hour. Drain beans in a

colander; rinse beans. In a slow cooker, stir together beans, lamb, broth, carrots, celery, onion, wine, garlic, bay leaves, rosemary, and pepper. Cover and cook on low for 8 to 10 hours or on high for 4 to 5 hours. Remove and discard bay leaves before serving.

Nutrition Info:

Per serving: 547 g water; 271 calories (19% from fat, 54% from protein, 27% from carb); 32 g protein; 5 g total fat; 2 g saturated fat; 2 g monounsaturated fat; 0 g polyunsaturated fat; 16 g carb; 5 g fiber; 3 g sugar; 269 mg phosphorus; 65 mg calcium; 4 mg iron; 159 mg sodium; 613 mg potassium; 3629 IU vitamin A; 0 mg ATE vitamin E; 4 mg vitamin C; 68 mg cholesterol

Vegetable Chili

Servings: 4 Servings

Ingredients:

- 1 cup (160 g) chopped onion
- 20 ounces (560 g) frozen mixed vegetables
- 1 can (14 ounces, or 400 g) no-salt-added diced tomatoes, undrained
- 1 cup (245 g) no-salt-added tomato sauce
- ½ cup (120 ml) water
- 1 tablespoon (7.5 g) chili powder

Directions:

1. Place onion in slow cooker. Place frozen vegetables in strainer; rinse with hot water to separate. Stir vegetables, undrained tomatoes, tomato sauce, water, and chili powder into onions. Cover and cook on low for 8 to 10 hours.

Nutrition Info:

Per serving: 327 g water; 152 calories (5% from fat, 16% from protein, 80% from carb); 6 g protein; 1 g total fat; 0 g saturated fat; 0 g monounsaturated fat; 0 g polyunsaturated fat; 31 g carb;

9 g fiber; 11 g sugar; 127 mg phosphorus; 89 mg calcium; 3 mg iron; 90 mg sodium; 731 mg potassium; 6932 IU vitamin A; 0 mg ATE vitamin E; 25 mg vitamin C; 0 mg cholesterol

Two-day Vegetable Soup

Servings: 8 Servings

Ingredients:

- 1 pound (455 g) beef chuck
- 2 cups (475 ml) low-sodium beef broth
- ½ cup (50 g) chopped celery
- ½ cup (80 g) chopped onion
- ½ teaspoon garlic powder
- 4 potatoes, diced
- 12 ounces (340 g) frozen mixed vegetables
- 4 ounces (115 g) mushrooms, sliced
- 1 cup (70 g) shredded cabbage
- 2 teaspoons (5 g) Salt-Free Seasoning Blend
- 1 tablespoon (1.3 g) parsley

Directions:

1. Day one: Place beef, broth, celery, and onion in slow cooker and cook on low for 8 to 10 hours. Cool. Remove meat from bones and chop. Skim fat from broth. Day two: Place meat and broth back in slow cooker. Add remaining ingredients and cook on low for 8 to 10 hours.

Nutrition Info:

Per serving: 283 g water; 313 calories (33% from fat, 19% from protein, 48% from carb); 15 g protein; 11 g total fat; 5 g saturated fat; 5 g monounsaturated fat; 1 g polyunsaturated fat; 38 g carb; 5 g fiber; 4 g sugar; 202 mg phosphorus; 42 mg calcium; 2 mg iron; 104 mg sodium; 849 mg potassium; 1902 IU vitamin A; 0 mg ATE vitamin E; 18 mg vitamin C; 40 mg cholesterol

Mexican Bean Soup

Servings: 8 Servings

Ingredients:

- 1 cup (160 g) chopped onion
- 1 can (14 ounces, or 400 g) no-salt-added diced tomatoes
- 2 cups (342 g) pinto beans, cooked or canned without salt
- 2 cups (344 g) black beans, cooked, or canned without salt
- 2 cups (512 g) kidney beans, cooked or canned without salt
- 1 pound (455 g) frozen corn
- 1½ cups (390 g) low-sodium salsa
- 2 tablespoons (15 g) Salt-Free Mexican Seasoning

Directions:

1. Combine all ingredients in slow cooker. Cover and cook on low 8 to 10 hours.

Nutrition Info:

Per serving: 209 g water; 355 calories (4% from fat, 23% from protein, 73% from carb); 21 g protein; 2 g total fat; 0 g saturated fat; 0 g monounsaturated fat; 1 g polyunsaturated fat; 67 g carb; 18 g fiber; 6 g sugar; 400 mg phosphorus; 118 mg calcium; 6 mg iron; 123 mg sodium; 1394 mg potassium; 304 IU vitamin A; 0 mg ATE vitamin E; 14 mg vitamin C; 0 mg cholesterol

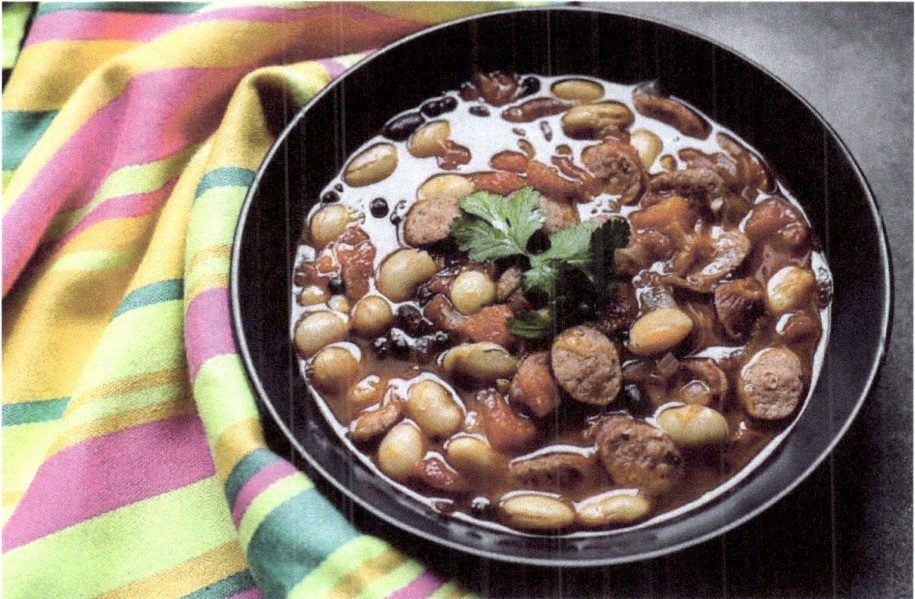

Bean Soup With Cornmeal Dumplings

Servings: 5 Servings

Ingredients:

- 2 cups (512 g) kidney beans, cooked or canned without salt
- 2 cups (344 g) black beans, cooked or canned without salt
- 3 cups (700 ml) low-sodium chicken broth
- 2 cups (360 ml) no-salt-added diced tomatoes
- 10 ounces (280 ml) frozen corn
- 1 cup (160 g) chopped onion
- 4 ounces (115 g) chopped green chilies
- 2 teaspoons chili powder
- ½ teaspoon minced garlic
- 2 tablespoons (15 g) Salt-Free Mexican Seasoning
- 1/3 cup (42 g) flour
- ¼ cup (35 g) cornmeal
- 1 teaspoon baking powder
- 2 tablespoons (28 ml) egg substitute
- 2 tablespoons (28 ml) skim milk

- 1 tablespoon (15 ml) olive oil

Directions:

1. Combine first 10 ingredients (through Mexican seasoning) in slow cooker. Cover and cook on low 8 to 10 hours. At the end of cooking time, turn cooker to high. Mix together flour, cornmeal, and baking powder. Combine egg, milk, and oil and stir into dry ingredients until just moistened. Drop dumplings by teaspoonful into soup. Cover and cook for 30 minutes.

Nutrition Info:

Per serving: 430 g water; 362 calories (12% from fat, 20% from protein, 68% from carb); 19 g protein; 5 g total fat; 1 g saturated fat; 2 g monounsaturated fat; 1 g polyunsaturated fat; 65 g carb; 17 g fiber; 6 g sugar; 349 mg phosphorus; 173 mg calcium; 6 mg iron; 324 mg sodium; 1034 mg potassium; 614 IU vitamin A; 4 mg ATE vitamin E; 25 mg vitamin C; 0 mg cholesterol

Minestrone

Servings: 10 Servings

Ingredients:

- 2 pounds (900 g) extra-lean ground beef
- 1 cup (160 g) chopped onion
- ½ teaspoon minced garlic
- 1 can (28 ounces, or 785 g) no-salt-added diced tomatoes
- 2 cups (512 g) kidney beans, cooked or canned without salt
- ½ cup (50 g) sliced celery
- 1½ cups (180 g) diced zucchini
- 2 cups (475 ml) low-sodium beef broth
- 2 teaspoons Italian seasoning

Directions:

1. Brown meat in skillet over medium-high heat. Drain. Combine meat and remaining ingredients in slow cooker. Cover and cook on low 8 to 10 hours.

Nutrition Info:

Per serving: 239 g water; 284 calories (50% from fat, 31% from protein, 19% from carb); 22 g protein; 16 g total fat; 6 g saturated fat; 7 g monounsaturated fat; 1 g polyunsaturated fat; 13 g carb; 5 g fiber; 3 g sugar; 213 mg phosphorus; 61 mg calcium; 4 mg iron; 107 mg sodium; 656 mg potassium; 168 IU vitamin A; 0 mg ATE vitamin E; 12 mg vitamin C; 63 mg cholesterol

Split Pea Soup

Servings: 6 Servings

Ingredients:

- ¾ cup (98 g) sliced carrots
- ½ cup (50 g) sliced celery
- 1 cup (160 g) chopped onion
- 1 parsnip, diced
- 1 pound (455 g) split peas, washed with stones removed
- 2 tablespoons (28 ml) olive oil
- 1 teaspoon thyme
- 4 cups (950 ml) low-sodium vegetable broth
- 4 cups (950 ml) water
- ½ teaspoon pepper
- 2 teaspoons chopped fresh parsley

Directions:

1. Combine all ingredients in slow cooker. Cover and cook on high 7 hours.

Nutrition Info:

Per serving: 434 g water; 193 calories (27% from fat, 21% from protein, 52% from carb); 10 g protein; 6 g total fat; 1 g saturated fat; 4 g monounsaturated fat; 1 g polyunsaturated fat; 26 g carb; 8 g fiber; 6 g sugar; 158 mg phosphorus; 93 mg calcium; 2 mg iron; 184 mg sodium; 629 mg potassium; 2790 IU vitamin A; 2 mg ATE vitamin E; 8 mg vitamin C; 0 mg cholesterol

Chicken And Rice Stew

Servings: About 6

Cooking Time: 8 Hrs

Ingredients:

- 2 med. Carrots
- 2 med. Leeks
- 1 cup Rice (uncooked)
- 12 oz Boneless Chicken (without skin)
- 1 tsp.Thyme
- ½ tsp. Rosemary
- 3 cans Chicken Broth (14 oz. each)
- 1 can cream of Mushroom Soup (10.75 oz.)
- ½ cup Onion (chopped)
- 1 clove Garlic

Directions:

1. Place all the ingredients in a slow cooker.
2. Cover the slow cooker.
3. Cook on low for 7 or 8 hrs. or on high for 4 hrs.
4. Serve hot.

Nutrition Info:

(Estimated Amount Per Serving): 245.5 Calories; 6.2 g Total Fat; 35.1 Cholesterol; 1761.1 mg Sodium; 21.2 Carbohydrates; 1.5 g Dietary Fiber; 25.2 g Protein

Turkey Zucchini Soup

Servings: 8 Servings

Ingredients:

- 8 ounces (225 g) frozen green beans
- 2 cups (240 g) thinly sliced zucchini
- 2 cups (280 g) chopped cooked turkey
- 1 cup (245 g) no-salt-added tomato sauce
- ½ cup (80 g) finely chopped onion
- 1 teaspoon Worcestershire sauce
- ½ teaspoon ground savory
- ¼ teaspoon black pepper
- 4 cups (950 ml) water
- 3 ounces (85 g) fat-free cream cheese, softened

Directions:

1. Thaw green beans by placing in strainer; run hot water over beans. In slow cooker, stir together beans, zucchini, turkey, tomato sauce, onion, Worcestershire sauce, savory, pepper, and water. Cover and cook on high for 2 to 3 hours. Blend about 1 cup (235 ml) hot soup liquid into cream cheese; return to cooker, stirring well. Heat through.

Nutrition Info:

Per serving: 238 g water; 106 calories (25% from fat, 49% from protein, 26% from carb); 13 g protein; 3 g total fat; 2 g saturated fat; 1 g monounsaturated fat; 0 g polyunsaturated fat; 7 g carb; 2 g fiber; 3 g sugar; 123 mg phosphorus; 44 mg calcium; 2 mg iron; 73 mg sodium; 377 mg potassium; 429 IU vitamin A; 19 mg ATE vitamin E; 15 mg vitamin C; 40 mg cholesterol

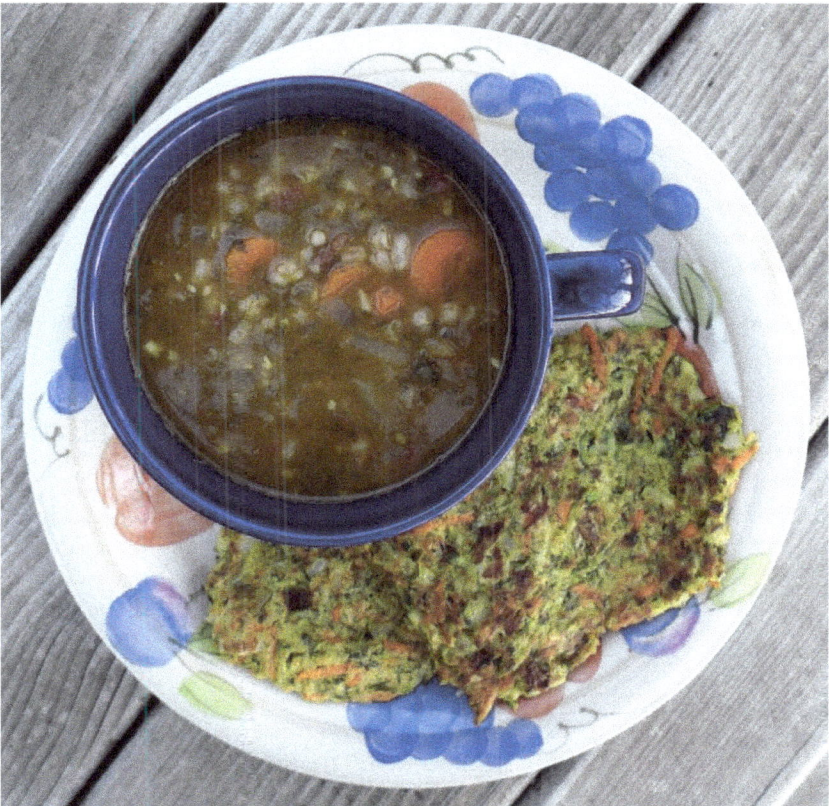

Black-eyed Pea Chili

Servings: 6 Servings

Ingredients:

- 1 cup (160 g) finely chopped onion
- 1 cup (130 g) finely chopped carrots
- 1 cup (150 g) finely chopped red pepper
- ½ teaspoon minced garlic
- 4 teaspoons (10 g) chili powder
- 1 teaspoon ground cumin
- 1 tablespoon (1 g) chopped cilantro
- 1 can (14 ounces, or 400 g) no-salt-added diced tomatoes
- 30 ounces (840 g) canned no-salt-added black-eyed peas, drained
- 4 ounces (115 g) diced green chilies
- 1 cup (235 ml) low-sodium vegetable broth

Directions:

1. Combine all ingredients in slow cooker. Cover and cook on low 6 to 8 hours or high 4 hours.

Nutrition Info:

Per serving: 279 g water; 242 calories (7% from fat, 23% from protein, 71% from carb); 15 g protein; 2 g total fat; 0 g saturated fat; 0 g monounsaturated fat; 1 g polyunsaturated fat; 45 g carb; 12 g fiber; 11 g sugar; 229 mg phosphorus; 96 mg calcium; 5 mg iron; 149 mg sodium; 913 mg potassium; 5101 IU vitamin A; 0 mg ATE vitamin E; 53 mg vitamin C; 0 mg cholesterol

Ham And Pea Soup

Servings: About 8

Cooking Time: 8 Hrs

Ingredients:

- 1 lb. Split Peas (dried)
- 1 cup sliced Celery
- 1 cup sliced Carrots
- 1 cup sliced Onion
- 2 cups chopped Ham (cooked)
- 8 cups Water

Directions:

1. Place all the ingredients in the slow cooker.
2. Cook on "high" for 4 hrs.
3. Serve hot.

Nutrition Info:

(Estimated Amount Per Serving): 118.6 Calories; 1.9 g Total Fat; 15.9 mg Cholesterol; 828.2 mg Sodium; 14.5 mg Carbohydrates; 5.1 g Dietary Fiber; 11.1 g Protein

Beef And Rice Stew

Servings: 6 Servings

Ingredients:

- ½ cup (30 g) sliced onion
- 1 pound (455 g) extra-lean ground beef
- ½ cup (93 g) uncooked long-grain rice
- 3 potatoes, diced
- 1 cup (100 g) diced celery
- 2 cups (508 g) no-salt-added kidney beans, drained
- ¼ teaspoon pepper
- ½ teaspoon chili powder
- 1 teaspoon Worcestershire sauce
- 1 cup (245 g) no-salt-added tomato sauce

Directions:

1. Brown onions and ground beef in skillet over medium-high heat. Drain. Layer beef mixture and remaining ingredients in slow cooker in order given. Cover and cook on low 6 hours or until potatoes and rice are cooked.

Nutrition Info:

Per serving: 301 g water; 458 calories (26% from fat, 22% from protein, 52% from carb); 25 g protein; 14 g total fat; 5 g saturated fat; 6 g monounsaturated fat; 1 g polyunsaturated fat; 59 g carb; 10 g fiber; 4 g sugar; 342 mg phosphorus; 70 mg calcium; 6 mg iron; 93 mg sodium; 1509 mg potassium; 289 IU vitamin A; 0 mg ATE vitamin E; 25 mg vitamin C; 52 mg cholesterol

Tomato Rice Soup

Servings: 4 Servings

Ingredients:

- 2 cups (360 g) no-salt-added diced tomatoes
- 1 can (6 ounces, or 170 g) no-salt-added tomato paste
- 2 cups (475 ml) water
- ½ cup (50 g) chopped celery
- 1 cup (160 g) minced onion
- 1 1/3 cups (245 g) rice

Directions:

1. Put tomatoes, tomato paste, water, celery, and onion into slow cooker. Cook on high for 1 hour and then add rice. Cook for 4 hours more.

Nutrition Info:

Per serving: 346 g water; 142 calories (3% from fat, 12% from protein, 84% from carb); 5 g protein; 1 g total fat; 0 g saturated fat; 0 g monounsaturated fat; 0 g polyunsaturated fat; 32 g carb; 4 g fiber; 10 g sugar; 95 mg phosphorus; 76 mg calcium; 3 mg iron; 73 mg sodium; 768 mg potassium; 847 IU vitamin A; 0 mg ATE vitamin E; 24 mg vitamin C; 0 mg cholesterol

Creamy Bean Soup

Servings: 6 Servings

Ingredients:

- 6 cups (1.4 L) water
- 2 cups (386 g) dried pinto beans
- ¼ cup (40 g) chopped onion
- ¼ teaspoon marjoram
- Dash black pepper
- 1 cup (235 ml) fat-free evaporated milk
- 1 tablespoon (8 g) flour

Directions:

1. In a saucepan, bring water and beans to boiling; reduce heat and simmer, covered, 1½ hours. Pour beans and cooking liquid into a bowl; cover and chill. Drain beans, reserving the cooking liquid. Transfer beans to slow cooker. Stir in onion, marjoram, and dash pepper. Add enough of the reserved cooking liquid to cover, about 2 cups (475 ml). Cover and cook on low for 12 to 14 hours. Turn to high. Slowly blend milk into flour; stir into beans in cooker. Cover and cook until thickened and bubbly, 10 to 15 minutes. Mash beans slightly, if desired.

Nutrition Info:

Per serving: 284 g water; 264 calories (3% from fat, 26% from protein, 71% from carb); 17 g protein; 1 g total fat; 0 g saturated fat; 0 g monounsaturated fat; 0 g polyunsaturated fat; 47 g carb; 10 g fiber; 6 g sugar; 351 mg phosphorus; 206 mg calcium; 3 mg iron; 64 mg sodium; 1052 mg potassium; 170 IU vitamin A; 50 mg ATE vitamin E; 5 mg vitamin C; 2 mg cholesterol

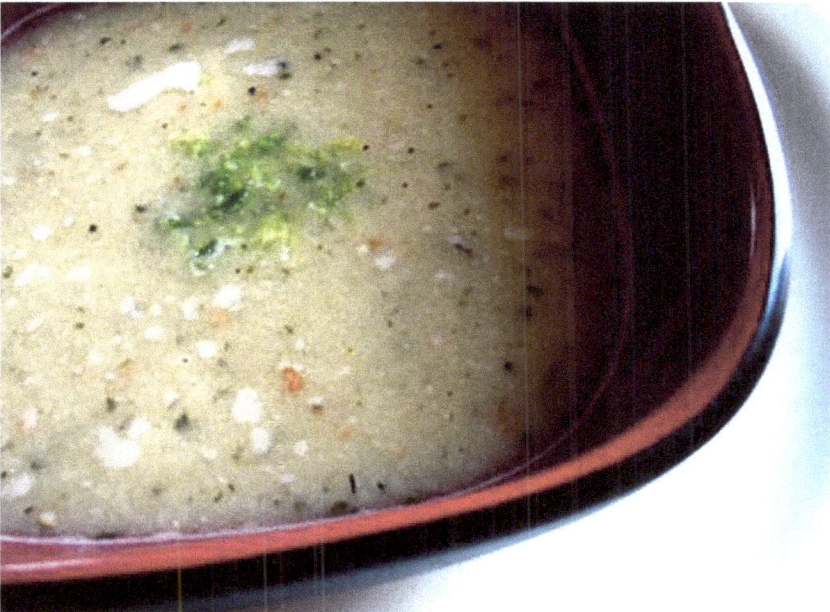

Veggie And Beef Soup

Servings: About 4

Cooking Time: 4 Hrs

Ingredients:

- 1 chopped Carrot
- 1 chopped Celery Rib
- ¾ l. Sirloin (ground)
- 1 cup Water
- ½ Butternut Squash (large)
- 1 clove Garlic
- ½ qrt Beef broth
- 7 ouncesdiced Tomatoes (unsalted)
- ½ tsp.Kosher Salt
- 1 tbsp. chopped Parsley
- ¼ tsp.Thyme (dried)
- ¼ tsp.Black Pepper (ground)
- ½ Bay Leaf

Directions:

1. Sauté all the vegetables in oil.
2. Push the vegetables to the side and place sirloin in the center.Sauté, using a spoon to crumble the meat.

68

3.   When cooked, combine with the vegetables on the sides of the pan.

4.   Now, pour rest of the ingredients in the slow cooker.

5.   Add in cooked meat and vegetables.

6.   Stir well.

7.   Cook on "low" for 3 hrs.

8.   Serve in soup bowls.

Nutrition Info:

(Estimated Amount Per Serving): 217 Calories; 7 g Total Fats; 53 mg Cholesterol; 728 mg Sodium; 17 mg Carbohydrates; 5 g Dietary Fiber; 22 g Protein

Vegetarian Vegetable Soup

Servings: 8 Servings

Ingredients:

- 2 cups (260 g) sliced carrot
- 1 pound (455 g) frozen green beans
- 1 pound (455 g) frozen corn
- 1 can (28 ounces, or 785 g) no-salt-added diced tomatoes
- 1 cup (160 g) chopped onion
- 2 cups (475 ml) low-sodium vegetable broth
- 1 tablespoon (15 ml) Worcestershire sauce

Directions:

1. Combine all ingredients in slow cooker. Cover and cook on low 8 to 10 hours.

Nutrition Info:

Per serving: 294 g water; 132 calories (14% from fat, 13% from protein, 73% from carb); 5 g protein; 2 g total fat; 1 g saturated fat; 1 g monounsaturated fat; 1 g polyunsaturated fat; 27 g carb; 6 g fiber; 7 g sugar; 124 mg phosphorus; 76 mg calcium; 2 mg iron;

101 mg sodium; 629 mg potassium; 6008 IU vitamin A; 0 mg ATE vitamin E; 30 mg vitamin C; 0 mg cholesterol

Sausage Soup

Servings: 6 Servings

Ingredients:

- 1 pound (455 g) kielbasa, sliced
- 6 cups (1.4 L) water
- 1 can (14 ounces, or 400 g) no-salt-added diced tomatoes
- ½ cup (50 g) sliced celery
- 1 cup (130 g) sliced carrots
- 1 cup (105 g) uncooked macaroni
- ½ teaspoon Salt-Free Seasoning Blend
- ½ teaspoon basil
- ½ teaspoon oregano
- 2 tablespoons (15 g) low-sodium onion soup mix

Directions:

1. Combine all ingredients in slow cooker. Cover and cook on low 8 to 10 hours.

Nutrition Info:

Per serving: 360 g water; 176 calories (54% from fat, 16% from protein, 30% from carb); 7 g protein; 11 g total fat; 4 g saturated

fat; 5 g monounsaturated fat; 1 g polyunsaturated fat; 13 g carb; 2 g fiber; 3 g sugar; 92 mg phosphorus; 59 mg calcium; 2 mg iron; 444 mg sodium; 333 mg potassium; 3713 IU vitamin A; 0 mg ATE vitamin E; 8 mg vitamin C; 25 mg cholesterol

Hominy Stew

Servings: 8 Servings

Ingredients:

- 1 can (28 ounces, or 785 g) no-salt-added diced tomatoes
- 4 ounces (115 g) canned chilies, chopped
- 4 cups (684 g) pinto beans, cooked or canned without salt
- 24 ounces (680 g) hominy, undrained
- 1 cup (160 g) chopped onion
- 2 cups (475 ml) water
- 2 tablespoons (15 g) Ranch Dressing Mix
- 2 tablespoons (15 g) Salt-Free Mexican Seasoning

Directions:

1. Combine all ingredients in slow cooker. Cover and cook on low 8 to 10 hours.

Nutrition Info:

Per serving: 204 g water; 658 calories (3% from fat, 17% from protein, 79% from carb); 29 g protein; 3 g total fat; 0 g saturated fat; 0 g monounsaturated fat; 1 g polyunsaturated fat; 134 g carb;

21 g fiber; 6 g sugar; 564 mg phosphorus; 155 mg calcium; 9 mg iron; 85 mg sodium; 1701 mg potassium; 134 IU vitamin A; 0 mg ATE vitamin E; 22 mg vitamin C; 0 mg cholesterol

Multi-bean Chili

Servings: 12 Servings

Ingredients:

- ½ pound (225 g) extra-lean ground beef
- ½ pound (225 g) sausage
- 1 cup (160 g) chopped onion
- 1 can (15 ounces, or 420 g) kidney beans, no-salt-added, undrained
- 1 can (15 ounces, or 420 g) black beans, no-salt-added, undrained
- 1 can (15 ounces, or 420 g) pinto beans, no-salt-added, undrained
- 1 can (14 ounces, or 400 g) no-salt-added stewed tomatoes, undrained
- 1 can (15 ounces, or 420 g) no-salt-added tomato sauce
- 2 tablespoons (15 g) Salt-Free Mexican Seasoning
- 3 tablespoons (45 g) brown sugar
- 3 tablespoons (23 g) chili powder

Directions:

1. Brown beef, sausage, and onion together in a nonstick skillet over medium-high heat. Combine meat mixture and remaining ingredients in large slow cooker. Mix well. Cook on low 8 to 10 hours.

Nutrition Info:

Per serving: 146 g water; 368 calories (24% from fat, 23% from protein, 52% from carb); 22 g protein; 10 g total fat; 4 g saturated fat; 4 g monounsaturated fat; 1 g polyunsaturated fat; 49 g carb; 14 g fiber; 8 g sugar; 330 mg phosphorus; 97 mg calcium; 5 mg iron; 204 mg sodium; 1119 mg potassium; 740 IU vitamin A; 0 mg ATE vitamin E; 12 mg vitamin C; 28 mg cholesterol

Chicken Rice Soup

Servings: 6 Servings

Ingredients:

- 1 pound (455 g) boneless skinless chicken breast, cut into 1-inch (2.5 cm) pieces
- 5 cups (1.2 L) low-sodium chicken broth
- 8 ounces (225 g) mushrooms, sliced
- ¾ cup (75 g) sliced celery
- ½ cup (65 g) sliced carrots
- ½ cup (93 g) uncooked long-grain rice
- ¼ cup (25 g) chopped scallions
- ½ teaspoon ground sage
- ¼ teaspoon black pepper

Directions:

1. Combine all ingredients in slow cooker. Cover and cook on low for 7 to 9 hours.

Nutrition Info:

Per serving: 318 g water; 149 calories (14% from fat, 62% from protein, 24% from carb); 23 g protein; 2 g total fat; 1 g saturated fat; 1 g monounsaturated fat; 1 g polyunsaturated fat; 9 g carb; 1

g fiber; 2 g sugar; 255 mg phosphorus; 31 mg calcium; 1 mg iron; 129 mg sodium; 569 mg potassium; 1908 IU vitamin A; 5 mg ATE vitamin E; 4 mg vitamin C; 44 mg cholesterol

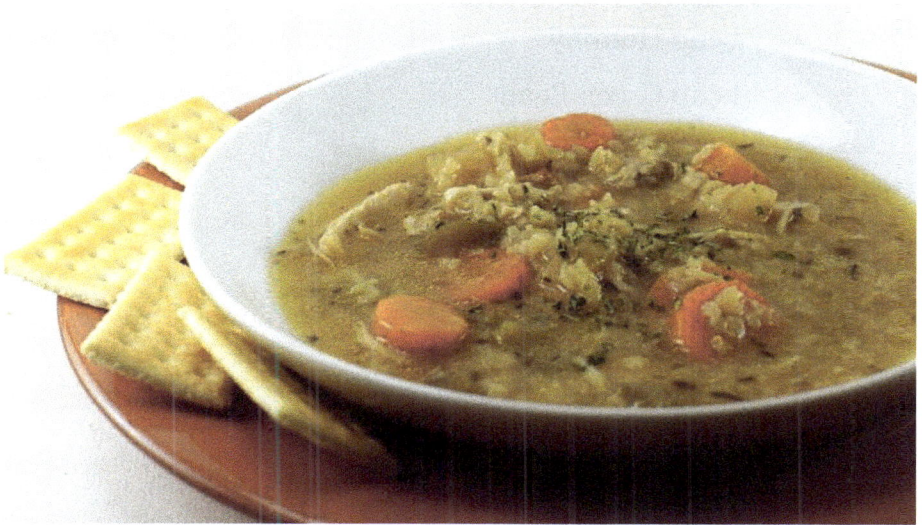

Vegetable Stew

Servings: 4-6

Cooking Time: 8 Hrs

Ingredients:

- 1 cup Corn
- 1 cup Hominy
- 1 cup Green Beans
- 1 canPeas (black eyed)
- 1 cup Lima Beans
- 1 cup chopped Carrots
- 1 cup chopped Celery
- 1 cup Onion
- 1 can Tomato Sauce (small)
- 2 cups Vegetable Broth
- 2 tbsp. Worcestershire Sauce

Directions:

1. Place all the ingredients in the slow cooker.
2. Cook on "low" for 8 hrs.
3. Serve hot.

Nutrition Info:

(Estimated Amount Per Serving): 186 Calories; 1.2 g Total Fat; 0 mg Cholesterol; 692.9 mg Sodium; 38.8 mg Carbohydrates; 10.3 g Dietary Fiber; 8.3 g Protein

Chicken And Wild Rice Soup

Ingredients:

- 2 tablespoons (28 g) unsalted butter
- ½ cup (80 g) wild rice
- 6 cups (1.4 L) low-sodium chicken broth
- ½ cup (80 g) minced onions
- ½ cup (50 g) minced celery
- ½ pound (225 g) butternut squash, peeled, seeded, and cut in ½-inch (1.3 cm) cubes
- 3 cups (420 g) chopped cooked chicken

Directions:

1. Melt butter in small skillet. Add rice and sauté for 10 minutes over low heat. Transfer to slow cooker. Add all remaining ingredients except chicken to cooker. Cover and cook on low 4 to 6 hours. One hour before serving, stir in chicken.

Nutrition Info:

Per serving: 260 g water; 154 calories (30% from fat, 39% from protein, 32% from carb); 15 g protein; 5 g total fat; 2 g saturated fat; 1 g monounsaturated fat; 1 g polyunsaturated fat; 12 g carb; 1 g fiber; 2 g sugar; 176 mg phosphorus; 35 mg calcium; 1 mg iron;

156 mg sodium; 358 mg potassium; 3162 IU vitamin A; 33 mg ATE vitamin E; 8 mg vitamin C; 47 mg cholesterol

Kale Verde

Servings: 6

Cooking Time: 6 Hrs

Ingredients:

- ¼ cup Olive Oil (extra virgin)
- 1 Yellow Onion (large)
- 2 cloves Garlic
- 2 ounces Tomatoes, dried
- 2 cups Yellow Potatoes (diced)
- 14 ounce Tomatoes (diced)
- 6 cups Chicken Broth
- White Pepper (ground)
- 1 pound o chopped Kale

Directions:

1. Sauté onion for 5 mins in oil.
2. Add the garlic and sauté again for 1 mins.
3. Transfer the sautéed mixture to the slow cooker.
4. Now, put the rest of the ingredients except pepper into the slow cooker.
5. Cook on "low" for 6 hrs.
6. Season with white pepper to taste.

7.   Serve hot in heated bowls

Nutrition Info:

(Estimated Amount Per Serving): 257 Calories; 22 g Total Fat; 3 mg Cholesterol; 239 mg Sodium; 27 mg Carbohydrates; 6 g Dietary Fiber; 14 g Protein

Brown Rice And Chicken Soup

Servings: About 4

Cooking Time: 4 Hrs

Ingredients:

- 1/3 cups Brown Rice
- 1 chopped Leek
- 1 sliced Celery Rib
- 1 ½ cups water
- ½ tsp. Kosher Salt
- ½ Bay Leaf
- 1/8 tsp. Thyme (dried)
- ¼ tsp. Black Pepper (ground)
- 1 tbsp. chopped Parsley
- ½ qrt Chicken Broth (low sodium)
- 1 sliced Carrot
- ¾ lb. of Chicken Thighs (skin and boneless)

Directions:

1. In a saucepan, boil 1 cup of water with ½ tsp. of Salt.
2. Add the rice.
3. Cook for 30 mins on medium flame.
4. Brown chicken pieces in the oil.

5. Transfer the chicken to a plate when done.

6. In same pan, sauté the vegetables for 3 mins.

7. Now, place the chicken pieces in the slow cooker. Add water and broth.

8. Cook on "low" for 3 hrs.

9. Now, add the rest of the ingredients, the rice last.

10. Cook again for 10 mins on "high".

11. After discarding Bay leaf, serve in soup bowls

Nutrition Info:

(Estimated Amount Per Serving): 208 Calories; 6 g Total Fats; 71 mg Cholesterol; 540 mg Sodium; 18 mg Carbohydrates; 2 g Dietary Fiber; 20 g Protein

Easy Cheesy Potato Soup

Servings: 6 Servings

Ingredients:

- 3 cups (700 ml) water
- 5 medium potatoes, diced finely
- 8 ounces (225 g) fat-free cream cheese, cubed
- ½ cup (80 g) chopped onion
- 1 teaspoon garlic powder
- ¼ teaspoon black pepper
- ½ teaspoon dill weed
- ½ cup (58 g) shredded Cheddar cheese

Directions:

1. Combine all ingredients in slow cooker. Cover and cook on high 4 hours, stirring occasionally.

Nutrition Info:

Per serving: 407 g water; 354 calories (27% from fat, 14% from protein, 59% from carb); 13 g protein; 11 g total fat; 7 g saturated fat; 3 g monounsaturated fat; 1 g polyunsaturated fat; 53 g carb; 6 g fiber; 4 g sugar; 306 mg phosphorus; 161 mg calcium; 3 mg iron; 203 mg sodium; 1503 mg potassium; 394 IU vitamin A; 97 mg ATE vitamin E; 28 mg vitamin C; 33 mg cholesterol

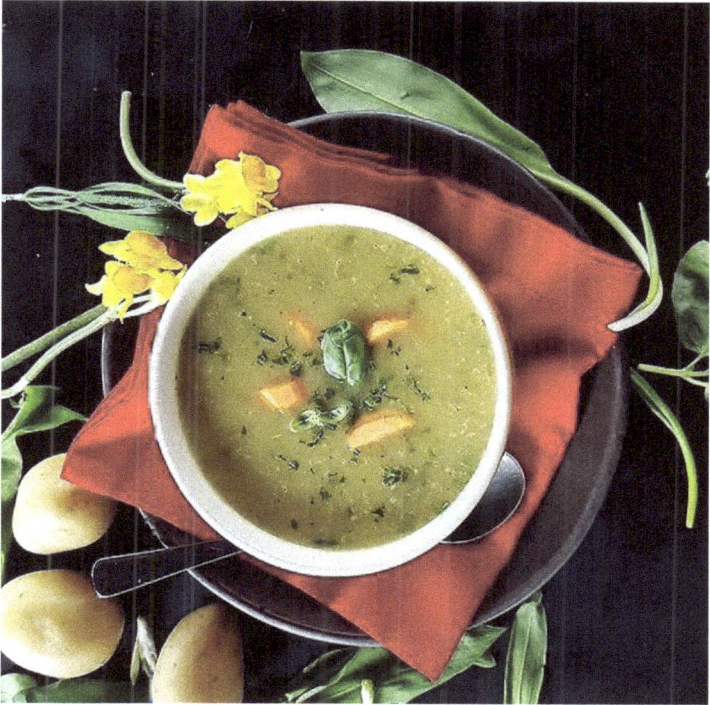

Mexican Chicken Soup

Servings: 8 Servings

Ingredients:

- 1 cup (160 g) chopped onion
- 1 cup (100 g) thinly sliced celery
- ½ teaspoon minced garlic
- 1 tablespoon (15 ml) oil
- 1½ pounds (680 g) boneless, skinless chicken breasts, cubed
- 3 cups (700 ml) low-sodium chicken broth
- 2 cups (520 g) low-sodium salsa
- 2 large potatoes, cubed
- 4 ounces (115 g) diced green chilies
- 4 ounces (115 g) Cheddar cheese, shredded

Directions:

1. Combine onions, celery, garlic, oil, chicken, and broth in slow cooker. Cover and cook on low 2½ hours until chicken is no longer pink. Add salsa, potatoes, chilies, and cheese and combine well. Cook on low 2 to 4 hours or until potatoes are fully cooked.

Nutrition Info:

Per serving: 326 g water; 262 calories (27% from fat, 40% from protein, 33% from carb); 27 g protein; 8 g total fat; 4 g saturated fat; 2 g monounsaturated fat; 1 g polyunsaturated fat; 21 g carb; 3 g fiber; 4 g sugar; 334 mg phosphorus; 155 mg calcium; 2 mg iron; 400 mg sodium; 925 mg potassium; 407 IU vitamin A; 42 mg ATE vitamin E; 17 mg vitamin C; 64 mg cholesterol

Beef And Black-eyed Pea Soup

Servings: 6 Servings

Ingredients:

- 1 pound (455 g) dry black-eyed peas
- 4 cups (950 ml) low-sodium beef broth
- 1 cup (130 g) sliced carrots
- 1 cup (160 g) chopped onion
- 2 pounds (900 g) beef round roast, cut into 1" cubes
- ½ teaspoon black pepper

Directions:

1. Combine all ingredients in slow cooker. Cover and cook on low 8 to 10 hours.

Nutrition Info:

Per serving: 359 g water; 324 calories (18% from fat, 53% from protein, 29% from carb); 42 g protein; 6 g total fat; 2 g saturated fat; 3 g monounsaturated fat; 0 g polyunsaturated fat; 23 g carb; 6 g fiber; 6 g sugar; 457 mg phosphorus; 73 mg calcium; 5 mg iron; 207 mg sodium; 1025 mg potassium; 3644 IU vitamin A; 0 mg ATE vitamin E; 5 mg vitamin C; 76 mg cholesterol

Italian Bean Soup

Servings: 6 Servings

Ingredients:

- 1 pound (455 g) dried mixed beans
- 1 cup (160 g) chopped onion
- 3 cups (700 ml) water
- 4 slices low-sodium bacon, cooked and crumbled
- 2 tablespoons (12 g) Italian seasoning
- 1 can (28 ounces, or 785 g) no-salt-added diced tomatoes

Directions:

1. Cook beans according to package directions until almost done. Drain. Combine beans and remaining ingredients in slow cooker. Cover and cook on low 8 to 10 hours.

Nutrition Info: Per serving: 276 g water; 317 calories (9% from fat, 26% from protein, 66% from carb); 21 g protein; 3 g total fat; 1 g saturated fat; 1 g monounsaturated fat; 1 g polyunsaturated fat; 54 g carb; 14 g fiber; 6 g sugar; 291 mg phosphorus; 248 mg calcium; 10 mg iron; 74 mg sodium; 1693 mg potassium; 226 IU vitamin A; 1 mg ATE vitamin E; 15 mg vitamin C; 6 mg cholesterol

Bean And Barley Soup

Servings: 10 Servings

Ingredients:

- 1 tablespoon (15 ml) olive oil
- 1 cup (160 g) chopped onion
- ¾ teaspoon minced garlic
- 24 ounces (680 g) no-salt-added great northern beans, undrained
- 4 cups (950 ml) low-sodium vegetable broth
- 4 cups (950 ml) water
- 1 cup (130 g) chopped carrots
- 1 cup (150 g) chopped green bell pepper
- ½ cup (50 g) chopped celery
- ½ cup (92 g) quick cooking barley
- ½ cup (30 g) chopped fresh parsley
- 2 bay leaves
- ½ teaspoon thyme
- ½ teaspoon black pepper
- 1 can (14 ounces, or 400 g) no-salt-added diced tomatoes, undrained

Directions:

1. Heat oil in a skillet over medium-high heat. Sauté onion and garlic until just soft. Combine onion mixture and remaining ingredients in slow cooker. Cook on low 8 to 10 hours. Discard bay leaves before serving.

Nutrition Info:

Per serving: 321 g water; 164 calories (13% from fat, 21% from protein, 66% from carb); 9 g protein; 2 g total fat; 0 g saturated fat; 1 g monounsaturated fat; 1 g polyunsaturated fat; 28 g carb; 6 g fiber; 3 g sugar; 167 mg phosphorus; 101 mg calcium; 2 mg iron; 83 mg sodium; 549 mg potassium; 2538 IU vitamin A; 1 mg ATE vitamin E; 23 mg vitamin C; 0 mg cholesterol

Borscht Stew

Servings: 6 Servings

Ingredients:

- 2 pounds (900 g) beef short ribs
- 2 cups (260 g) sliced carrots
- 1½ cups (225 g) turnips, peeled, sliced, and cut in strips
- 2 cups (450 g) beets, peeled, sliced, and cut in strips
- 1 medium onion, sliced
- 1 cup (100 g) sliced celery
- 3 cups (700 ml) water
- 1 can (6 ounces, or 170 g) no-salt-added tomato paste
- 1 tablespoon (13 g) sugar
- 1 tablespoon (15 ml) vinegar
- ¼ teaspoon pepper
- 4 cups (360 g) cabbage, cut in wedges

Directions:

1. In a large skillet over medium heat, slowly brown the short ribs on all sides. Drain off the excess fat. Place the sliced carrots, turnips, beets, onion, and celery in slow cooker. Place short ribs on top of the vegetables.

97

Stir together the water, tomato paste, sugar, vinegar, and pepper; mix well. Pour the mixture over the ribs. Cover and cook on low for 10 to 12 hours. Just before serving, skim the excess fat from stew. Fifteen minutes before serving, cook cabbage wedges in a 3-quart (2.8 L) saucepan in a large amount of boiling salted water until tender, 10 to 12 minutes. Drain cabbage well. Transfer ribs, vegetables, and cabbage to individual soup bowls.

Nutrition Info:

Per serving: 463 g water; 364 calories (39% from fat, 35% from protein, 26% from carb); 32 g protein; 16 g total fat; 7 g saturated fat; 7 g monounsaturated fat; 1 g polyunsaturated fat; 24 g carb; 6 g fiber; 15 g sugar; 372 mg phosphorus; 97 mg calcium; 6 mg iron; 292 mg sodium; 1297 mg potassium; 7756 IU vitamin A; 0 mg ATE vitamin E; 40 mg vitamin C; 89 mg cholesterol

Chicken And Sweet Potato Stew

Servings: About 5

Cooking Time: 5 Hrs

Ingredients:

- 6 Chicken Thighs
- 2 pounds peeled and sliced Sweet Potatoes
- ½ pound sliced Mushrooms
- 6 Shallots (halved)
- 4 peeled cloves Garlic
- 1 cup White Wine (dry)
- 2 tsp. chopped Rosemary
- 1 tsp. Salt
- ½ tsp Pepper (ground)
- ½ tbsp. Vinegar (white wine)

Directions:

1. Place all the ingredients in the slow cooker.
2. Cook on "low" for 5 hrs.
3. Serve hot after removing bones.

Nutrition Info:

(Estimated Amount Per Serving)300 Calories; 6 g Total Fat; 50 mg Cholesterol; 520 mg Sodium; 38 mg Carbohydrates; 5 g Dietary Fiber; 18 g Protein

Pea Soup

Servings: About 8

Cooking Time: 8 Hrs

Ingredients:

- 16 oz. Split Peas (dried)
- 1 cup chopped Baby Carrots
- 1chopped Onion (white)
- 3 Bay Leaves
- 10 oz. cubed Turkey Ham
- 4 cubes Chicken Bouillon
- 7 cups Water

Directions:

1. Rinse and drain peas.
2. Place all the ingredients in the slow cooker.
3. Cook on "low" for 8 hrs. Serve hot.

Nutrition Info:

(Estimated Amount Per Serving): 122.7 Calories; 2 g Total Fat; 24 mg Cholesterol; 780.6 mg Sodium; 15 mg Carbohydrates; 5.2 g Dietary Fiber; 11.8 g Protein

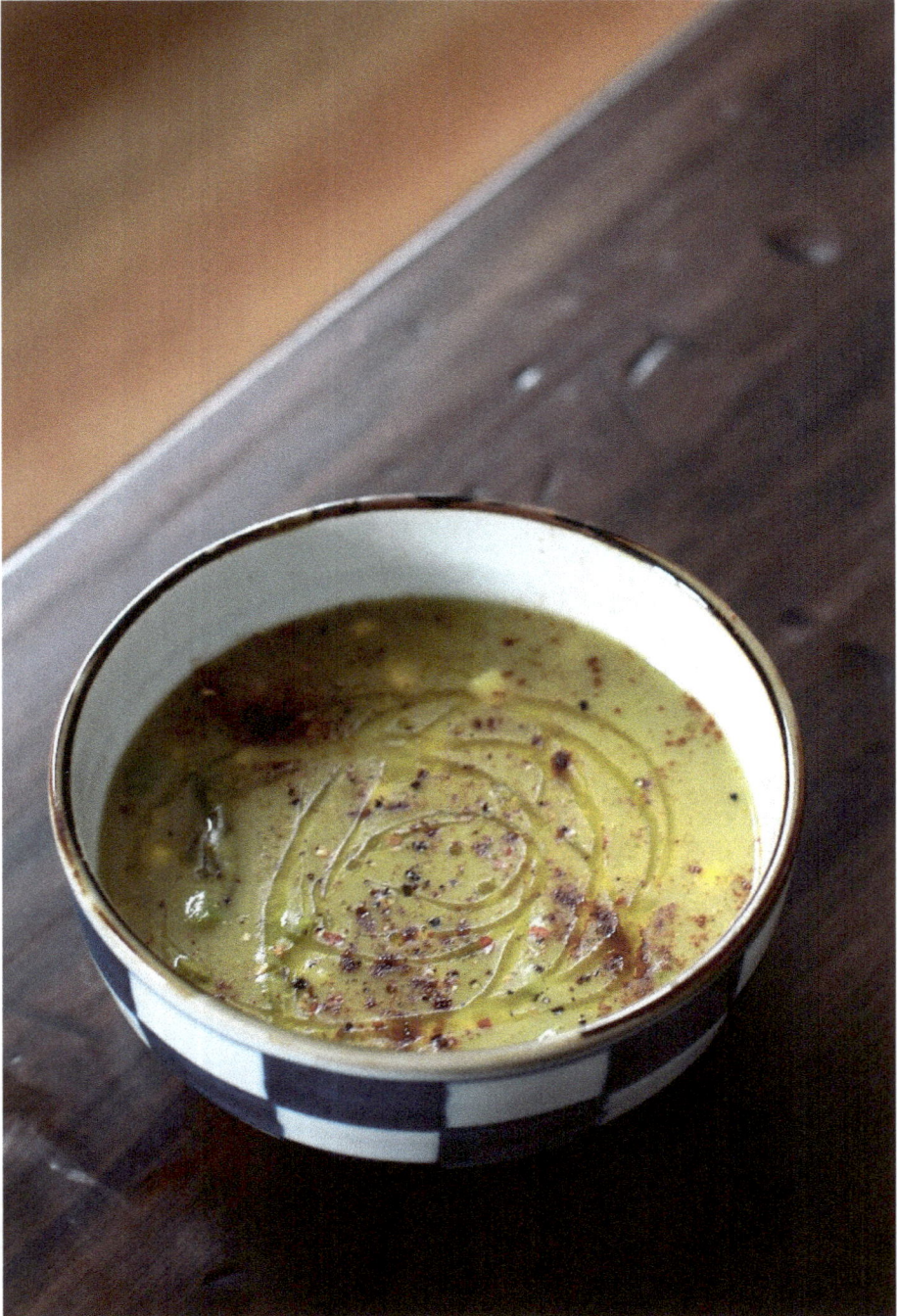

4-WEEK MEAL PLAN

Week 1

Monday

Breakfast: Tofu Frittata

Lunch: Pork Chops In Beer

Dinner: Stewed Tomatoes

Tuesday

Breakfast: Tapioca

Lunch: Creamy Beef Burgundy

Dinner: Oregano Salad

Wednesday

Breakfast: Fruit Oats

Lunch: Smothered Steak

Dinner: Black Beans With Corn Kernels

Thursday

Breakfast: Grapefruit Mix

Lunch: Pork For Sandwiches

Dinner: Stuffed Acorn Squash

Friday

Breakfast: Berry Yogurt

Lunch: Cranberry Pork Roast

Dinner: Greek Eggplant

Saturday
Breakfast: Soft Pudding
Lunch: Pan-asian Pot Roast
Dinner: Thyme Sweet Potatoes

Sunday
Breakfast: Black Beans Salad
Lunch: Short Ribs
Dinner: Barley Vegetable Soup

Week 2

Monday
Breakfast: Carrot Pudding
Lunch: French Dip
Dinner: Butter Corn

Tuesday
Breakfast: Apple Cake
Lunch: Italian Roast With Vegetables
Dinner: Orange Glazed Carrots

Wednesday
Breakfast: Almond Milk Barley Cereals
Lunch: Honey Mustard Ribs
Dinner: Cinnamon Acorn Squash

Thursday

Breakfast: Cashews Cake

Lunch: Pizza Casserole

Dinner: Glazed Root Vegetables

Friday

Breakfast: Artichoke Frittata

Lunch: Hawaiian Pork Roast

Dinner: Stir Fried Steak, Shiitake And Asparagus

Saturday

Breakfast: Mexican Eggs

Lunch: Apple Cranberry Pork Roast

Dinner: Cilantro Brussel Sprouts

Sunday

Breakfast: Stewed Peach

Lunch: Swiss Steak

Dinner: Italian Zucchini

Week 3

Monday

Breakfast: Lamb Cassoule t

Lunch: Glazed Pork Roast

Dinner: Cilantro Parsnip Chunks

Tuesday

Breakfast: Fruited Tapioca

Lunch: Swiss Steak In Wine Sauce

Dinner: Corn Casserole

Wednesday

Breakfast: Baby Spinach Shrimp Salad

Lunch: Italian Pork Chops

Dinner: Pilaf With Bella Mushrooms

Thursday

Breakfast: Coconut And Fruit Cake

Lunch: Italian Pot Roast

Dinner: Italian Style Yellow Squash

Friday

Breakfast: Apple And Squash Bowls

Lunch: Beef With Horseradish Sauce

Dinner: Stevia Peas With Marjoram

Saturday

Breakfast: Slow Cooker Chocolate Cake

Lunch: Oriental Pot Roast

Dinner: Broccoli Rice Casserole

Sunday

Breakfast: Fish Omelet

Lunch: Barbecued Ribs

Dinner: Italians Style Mushroom Mix

Week 4

Monday
Breakfast: Brown Cake
Lunch: Ham And Scalloped Pota toes
Dinner: Broccoli Casserole

Tuesday
Breakfast: Stevia And Walnuts Cut Oats
Lunch: Pork And Pineapple Roast

Wednesday
Breakfast: Walnut And Cinnamon Oatmeal
Lunch: Barbecued Brisket
Dinner: Dinner: Slow Cooker Lasagna

Thursday
Breakfast: Tender Rosemary Sweet Potatoes
Lunch: Barbecued Short Ribs
Dinner: Brussels Sprouts Casserole

Friday
Breakfast: Orange And Maple Syrup Quinoa
Lunch: Beer-braised Short Ribs
Dinner: Pasta And Mushrooms

Saturday
Breakfast: Vanilla And Nutmeg Oatmeal
Lunch: Lamb Stew
Dinner: Onion Cabbage

Sunday

Breakfast: Pecans Cake

Lunch: Barbecued Ham

Dinner: Cheese Broccoli

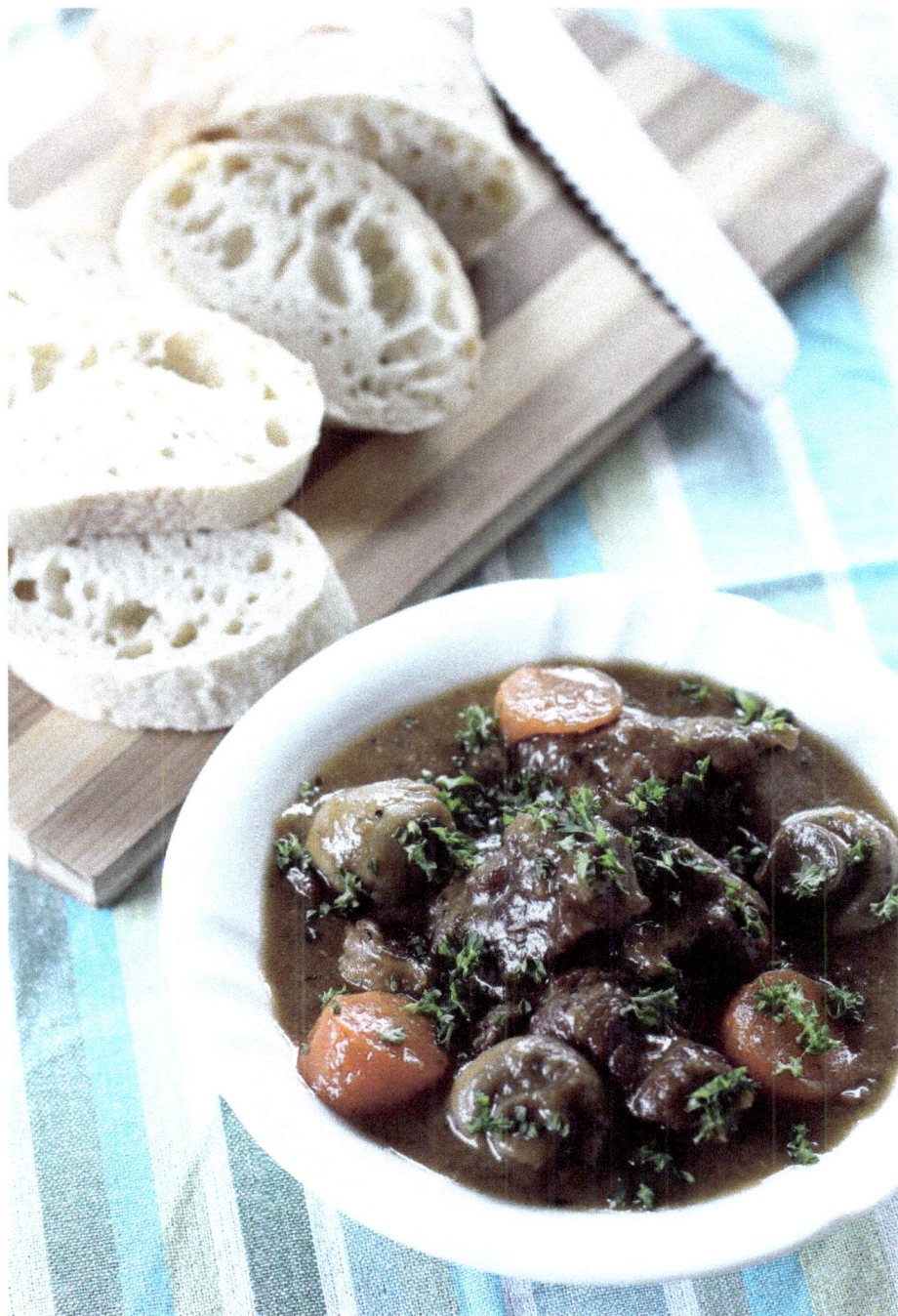

Ingram Content Group UK Ltd.
Milton Keynes UK
UKHW020602250423
420741UK00001B/22